Tourette's Syndrome

Our Story,
Everything We Wish We Were Told,
and Hints We Learned Along the Way

~

Pamela Smerglia

PUBLISH AMERICA

PublishAmerica
Baltimore

First printing

ISBN: 1-60441-275-5
PUBLISHED BY PUBLISHAMERICA, LLLP
www.publishamerica.com
Baltimore

Printed in the United States of America

Tourette's Syndrome

Our Story,
Everything We Wish We Were Told,
and Hints We Learned Along the Way

~

Pamela Smerglia

There are so many people who have made this book possible, and so many who have supported Dyllon and our family through trials and tribulations. To Dr. Mark Braunstein, I humbly thank you for your patience, guidance, support, and your nature in helping Dyllon and our family deal with, understand and live with a child with a disability. To Mrs. Regan Thaw, I owe you a debt of gratitude for your caring and supportive nature. You made the difference that first day in your office. Your suggestions, your ideas, and overall caring and willing attitude will never be forgotten.

To Dyllon, I thank you for being such a wonderful child. You are so creative and amazing. You give everything your best effort. Despite any challenges that come your way, you will always succeed. Keep your faith and ideals that life can be lived through rose-colored glasses.

Last but certainly not least, to Jason, my wonderful and supportive husband. You have been there when I needed an encouraging word and to push me through when I couldn't find my way. You have been my rock and biggest fan. Thank you for your years of support and understanding; I could not have done this without you.

Chapter 1

Our Story

As parents we naturally want our children to be "normal," to fit in, to be successful, socially and academically. What is "normal," and when do we get our children professional help? Through my story, I hope to help parents and educators understand that children with Tourette's syndrome are "normal," with a few special attributes.

I can remember the first time I thought something was "wrong" with my (at the time) seven-year-old son, Dyllon. For what seemed like an eternity but was actually months, Dyllon seemed to be angry, frustrated, and mad at the world, all the time. He was in first grade, and excelling academically, but socially he was far behind. I can remember dreading the magic hour of 3:00 p.m., when the school bus would pull up in front of the house. Not because I did not want to hear about Dyllon's day at school, but because I didn't know what kind of mood he would be in, or how many "rages" we would have that day. I say rages, because that is exactly what they were. Dyllon could be happy one minute, and screaming like a mad monkey the next. Anything could trigger the rages; it could be his brother touched him, or his shoe came untied, or anything that seemed insignificant to us, was a major crisis to him. We tried all sorts of punishments, taking away video game privileges, taking away t.v. time, grounding to his room, extra chores, we even took everything out of his room, except his bed and clothes, thinking that would work. We tried everything, and nothing seemed to help him or us for that matter. Now while all this was going on, Dyllon was having "tics," but we didn't know them to be "tics" at the time. We just thought they were annoying "habits" that Dyllon had. He would blink his eyes nonstop, clear his throat, whistle all the time, burp all the time—there were several, and we thought these were annoying habits that all children go through. During this period of time, the rages, and "habits," were accompanied by other "habits," like washing his hands every fifteen minutes, never letting his food touch other food on his plate, the tags in his shirt had to all be cut out because they annoyed him, his socks had to "fit" just right, his bed sheets had to be so tightly pulled under the bed you could bounce a quarter off it—all these things we, as his parents, found annoying. Later we would learn the things we called "habits" were called tics, and the "habits" we thought were annoying were called obsessions. The outbursts we called rages were just that, rages.

I remember the day that I called for help; it is burned into my memory forever. Everything was going smoothly, Dyllon was getting ready for school, Daddy was getting ready for work, and then the dark clouds moved in and the thunder started beaming down. The dark clouds being Dyllon's rage, and the thunder being the screaming and yelling. Dyllon was so upset, I will go so far as to say distraught, because the little red line on his socks was not even. Now that would seem like a little thing, easily remedied; not for Dyllon, however. He began melting down, throwing his shoes, and anything else he could get his hands on, screaming and yelling, he was out of control. I literally had to physically restrain him, for fear he would hurt himself. He was crying because he couldn't understand why his socks wouldn't fit, and I was crying because I didn't know why my child was acting like he was. I yelled for his father to come, and after some time of holding Dyllon, he calmed down, and I knew we needed help. Now here is the kicker, Dyllon had no recollection of the events that had just taken place. We decided to keep him home from school and make phone calls to get an appointment with a psychologist. That was the beginning of our understanding of Tourette's syndrome and associated disorders.

Now Jason, Dyllon's father, was so against psychology; he had the same thought that many people do, that psychology is bunk, it does not work, psychology is for "crazy" people, "shrinks" are a waste of money. So when he wanted to seek help for our son, I knew he was just as desperate for answers as I was.

We were very fortunate to get an appointment the next day. We told Dyllon that we were taking him to see a "special" friend to help him and us understand why he was acting like he was. I tell you, it was the best decision we ever could haves made; my only regret is I didn't make that call six months earlier.

So the big day was here. I thought our prayers have been answered, and someone is going to tell me what is wrong with my son, what I was doing wrong, what I could do better, I was going to get my "miracle cure in an hour." Boy, was I wrong. We drove an hour to the doctor's office. It was a nice drive through the mountains of southeast Colorado. It was a nice, warm fall day. The sun was shining, the views of the landscape were breathtaking. We didn't talk the whole trip there. I was in my own world, running things through my head, like what are they going to tell me, what is Dyllon going to tell them, is this really going to help, all those things that you wonder when you go to a psychologist's office. Jason was driving, and as usual, was quiet; I couldn't tell you what was in his mind, but I reckon it was the same thoughts I was having. Dyllon was in the back seat, playing his Nintendo Gameboy, so I know what he was thinking, "can I win this game."

We arrived at the office and walked in. It was a two-level office, shared by many different specialities of doctors. It smelled like a fresh linen closet, not like a sterile environment. We walked up the stairs to the psychologist's office and checked in. The secretary was nice. She handed me a stack of papers to fill out, and smiled that smile that tells you everything is going to be okay, without saying words. I retreated to the couch that was surrounded by chairs and tables with magazines covering the tops of them. I had the task of filling out the paperwork, while Jason thumbed blindly through the magazines, and Dyllon was still playing his game. As I was answering the questions on Dyllon's medical history and family history, I couldn't help but think this was somehow my fault. Like I did this to my child, the guilt overwhelmed me, and I struggled to get through the paperwork in tears.

From the corner of my eye, I saw this person coming towards us. She was thin, young and pretty. She spoke in a soft voice, and introduced herself. Her name is Reagan Thaw. She shook Dyllon's hand and asked him if it was alright if she talked to his parents first, and then she would spend some time with him. Dyllon didn't care; that meant he had more time to play his game. Jason and I followed Regan to her office, which was surprisingly inviting. It was full of games for kids, and soft couches that swallowed you up as you sat down. She began by telling us a little about her, her education, her philosophy on talking to children and the different techniques of "reaching" the root of the problem. She made you feel comfortable from the beginning, and for first-timers like us, that was important to us.

We began explaining all the things Dyllon was going through, and again the tears came on. She understood my guilt and sadness, and expressed that this is not my fault, and handed me tissues. We then retreated back out to the waiting area, and it was Dyllon's turn. He went in and had a nice chat with Regan, for which seemed like again another eternity, but was actually 30 minutes. Regan and Dyllon came out, and she asked to speak with us again, and Dyllon sat and played his game again. Jason and I were so far pleased with what was going on. Back in Regan's office, she assured us that there was hope for progress, and that Dyllon was an exceptional young man, who understood what was going on, more than we knew. He told her he didn't like feeling the way he was feeling, and was sad about the rages, but he couldn't control them. She recommended that Dyllon have weekly appointments with her, and that we also consult with another doctor in the office, a psychiatrist, who happened to be her husband, Dr. Mark Braunstein. Jason and I felt for the first time there was some hope, and we thanked her for seeing us and making us feel comfortable, and for making Dyllon feel comfortable. We made the appointments and left. The drive home was different than the drive there. I was not crying, I was excited that Dyllon was going to get the help that we could not give him.

We were again fortunate enough to have an appointment a week later with Dr. Mark, the psychiatrist. This time the hour trip was not full of dread, it was full of hope. Again we made the climb to the second level and checked in, and again the secretary had her usual comforting smile. We sat down and waited for Dr. Mark, when suddenly a HUGE dog came from down the hall. He was a sweet dog, and ran right over to Dyllon for love. From down the hall we could hear "Sage, come here," from this voice of a man, again, soft spoken. We thought it would come from a rather short man, but to our surprise, the voice calling Sage was from a rather tall young man (to this day I still don't know how tall he is). He came over to us and introduced himself, and told us to come back to his office. His office was different than Regan's office. It was full of medical books and dog toys, two couches, a desk and chair. More like a doctor's office, but still warm and inviting. Mark introduced himself and told us about himself as well. After looking over Regan's notes, and discussing things with us, he talked about bipolar disorder. That Dyllon's behavior mirrored all the signs of bipolar. We discussed all the treatment options, and decided medication would be the best. Mark was so patient with us, he explained all the side effects from medicine, and that only time will tell. We talked about the medicine with Dyllon, and he said, "Let's try it, it might help." Talk about an intelligent child.

The medicine, boy was that a big decision for us. We said we would never medicate our child, but couldn't let him to continue living with the way things were, because in reality, he wasn't really living a full life. Our first round of medication trials was Zyprexa, and it seemed to work, for a while anyway. Things did get better, less rages; we still had them, but they were not as intense and weren't as violent as before the medication. When Dyllon first started the medication, we noticed that his tics had become more noticeable, even to Dyllon. His first tic that we noticed, that was there all the time, was a neck tic. He rolled his neck in a snake motion. When we mentioned it to Dr. Mark, he became concerned that something else might be going on, so we were keeping an eye on it, and making note of other tics that presented themselves. Now keep in mind, we still didn't know at this time Dyllon had Tourette's syndrome.

After some months on Zyprexa, Dyllon was maxed out on the dosage he could be taking for his age and weight, and we were back to having rages all the time, and finding ourselves feeling desperate to help Dyllon. After we had so much success with medication, to feel like we were back at the beginning was devastating. Dr. Mark suggested a new medication, and some tests be run. We made appointments for an EEG and MRI. The EEG was no big deal, a cap on the head, and Dyllon slept for an hour, easy stuff. The MRI was a whole new ball of wax. Dyllon was taking Seroquel at the time, and it helped tremendously with the behavior issues. He was back to being a fun-loving, happy child. He was excelling in school, and of course we still had the obsessions with perfection. He didn't like to get dirty, handwriting had to be perfect, size and shape, socks had to fit one way, and no tags in the shirts.

Okay so back to the MRI. We made the appointment and waited. It was two weeks before we could get him in. The morning of the appointment, everything was going well, Dyllon was stable, in a good mood, I thought this was going to be cake! I was wrong. We got ready to go in to the MRI machine, and Dyllon did really good, until it was time to put him into the tube. He panicked and became claustrophobic. Who knew this would happen? It was another phobia that we didn't know about until we were in the situation. Obviously, we could not do the MRI that day, so we left. I was so angry at Dyllon for not going through with the MRI, and I was feeling so guilty for being angry. We did make another appointment, and talked to Dyllon about it. Regan and Mark talked to Dyllon about it, and we felt like this time he would do it. We gave him extra medicine, to calm him, and he did do it. It took some coaxing and patient talking, but he made it through. Of course the bribe of a new toy did not hurt.

Now was the big wait. Waiting for tests results and still not knowing what was going on with your child was a nightmare. We continued with the therapy sessions with

Regan and Mark, and some medicine changes, and things were great. Dyllon still had the tics and the obsessions, but we did not have the rages. He was stable, and that was enough for us.

Two weeks went by, and the results from the MRI came in. We were on pins and needles. They were inconclusive, but we did know that he was not having seizures. That was a relief in itself, but still no answers. This was a double-edge sword. On one hand we had good news, and on the other hand we still didn't have answers. So, the next step was a pediatric neurologist. We waited four months for that appointment, but it was worth it in the end.

In the meantime, Dyllon continued to make great progress, he learned techniques to calm the frustration, and we learned how to "deal" with him. We knew Dyllon had all the symptoms of Tourette's, but we didn't have a diagnosis, that would come later. We went through the "waxing" and "waning" of the tics, different tics, and through many hours of research, learned what things Dyllon was doing were actually tics.

Finally the big day. Again we wanted answers but learned from the first time that answers don't always come immediately. That is hard to swallow when you want the best for your child and you're as impatient as I am. Well the day began at 5:00 a.m. We had our best friends come over to stay with our other children, and we got on the road for a three-hour trip. It had snowed the night before, and the roads were not that bad, but I forgot the mountains would be worse than the main highway, and they were. What was supposed to be a three-hour trip turned into an eight-hour trip. I didn't care though; we waited four months for an appointment, and nothing was going to stop us from going. We were literally ten minutes away, and already thirty minutes late. I called my pastor at church, and asked them to call the hospital (I didn't have the number with me) and explain that we were in traffic because of the snow, and would be there as soon as possible. Well, three hours later, we made it.

It was at the University Hospital, and typical hospital setting, that sterile smell, and that feeling of doom and gloom. To my surprise, they kept an appointment open for us, and saw us as soon as we got there. The pediatric neurologist was an older woman, slender, and very pretty. She introduced herself and looked over Dyllon's medical records that had been sent. Then she talked to Dyllon and asked him how he was feeling and what he felt about all the "movements" he was doing. He explained to her that he knew he was doing it, but couldn't stop it. She then asked us about the different things Dyllon had been doing. It was clear Dyllon had Tourette's syndrome. I am telling you, it was like a million-pound weight had been lifted off my shoulders, like the heavens opened up and the angels were singing. The doctor explained Tourette's syndrome in detail; she spent an hour with us just explaining it and answering our questions. I know that doctor was busy, but she treated us like we were her only patient. She was not condescending, she was compassionate and understanding, and made sure we understood everything before we left. I have to tell you, that was the best two hours of my life. I finally had the answers I was looking for, I finally could put a "name" to what my child was experiencing. Suddenly everything made sense, and then the guilt came.

The drive home was a guilt-ridden one for me. I was so upset over the things we had done and said, and the whole time Dyllon had no control over what he was doing. The doctor had given us some pamphlets, and I read them cover to cover on the way home.

That was six months ago, and Dyllon is doing exceptionally well. We have the tics, we have the obsessions, but we wouldn't have it any other way. We have a better understanding of Tourette's, and a better understanding of how to deal with a child that has Tourette's syndrome.

Through this book, we hope to help other parents that are new and those that are not new to Tourette's, by telling them everything we wished we had been told, besides the medical lingo. We wish we had been told the everyday life stuff when Dyllon was diagnosed with Tourette's syndrome.

Chapter 2

What Is Tourette's Syndrome?

When we hear of person having Tourette's syndrome, the first thing that most people think of is a person, child or adult, that has uncontrollable outbursts of cursing and foul language. For 90 percent of the population that is diagnosed with Tourette's syndrome, that is a common mistake. They don't lash out with colorful four-letter words at strangers on the street. They are people who have repeated involuntary movements and uncontrollable vocal (phonic) sounds called tics. In a few cases, such tics can include inappropriate words and phrases.

Tourette's is a disorder named for Dr. Georges Gilles de la Tourette, the pioneering French neurologist who first described an 86-year-old noblewoman with the condition in 1885.

The symptoms of TS generally appear before the individual is 18 years old. Tourette's syndrome can affect people of all ethnic groups. The natural course of Tourette's syndrome will vary from patient to patient. The symptoms can range from very mild to quite severe, with the majority of cases falling into the mild category.

What are Tourette's syndrome tics? How do I know what they are, and how do I know they are tics? First let's begin by defining tics. Tics are rapid movements or sounds that are repeated over and over again for no reason. Although Tourette's syndrome tics have been described as rapid or sudden, not all are. Some tics are held or tonic movements involving freezing in one position for a few seconds. A person with Tourette's syndrome cannot control the movements or sounds. With children it is important to understand that the child may not be aware of their tics, and even if they are aware, they may have no ability to suppress them. Try not to blink…this will help you understand how hard it is to stop a Tourette tic. Tourette's syndrome tics are often worse when a person feels stressed, tired, or anxious. Other factors that affect tics can include medicines, heat, cold, and food or environmental allergies.

There are two categories of Tourette's syndrome tics: simple and complex. Simple tics are a sudden movement that involves a small amount of muscle groups. They are often repetitive. Simple motor tics are movements involving one group of muscles, for example, eye blinking, face grimacing, shoulder shrugging, head turning, neck movements, or tongue protrusion.

Simple vocal tics are meaningless noises that can be annoying, such as grunting, sniffing, clearing the throat, squeaking, whistling, or any other vocal sound. These are not to be confused with inappropriate outbursts of words or phrases, that will come later in definition.

Complex tics are distinct, coordinated patterns of successive movement involving several muscle groups. Complex motor tics are patterns of movement that resemble normal motor tasks or gestures, like jumping, smelling, touching things, touching other people, smelling things, smelling fingers, or smelling shoes.

Complex vocal tics include meaningful syllables, words, or phrases. Often but not always vocal tics occur at points of speech transition, such as the beginning of a sentence, or phrase transition. They may have an alteration in speech volume, slur a phrase, overemphasize a word or take on an accent.

Tourette's syndrome tics only require treatment when they interfere with the life or quality of life of the person living with Tourette's.

Chapter 3

Common Tics of Tourette's Syndrome

Tic periods can last from a few days to a few weeks to a few months. This list is not all inclusive, but gives you a great guideline for distinguishing tics.

Abdominal jerking
Abdominal tension
Animal sounds
Ankle flexing
Arm squeezing, jerking, flexing, flapping, extending
Banging
Barking
Belching
Bending
Blowing on fingers or objects

Change in voice tone, tempo, volume
Chewing on clothes, or other objects
Clicking
Coughing
Clearing throat
Clapping
Eye blinking
Eye rolling
Finger movements
Foot dragging
Foot shaking
Foot tapping
Funny expressions
Gasping
Grimacing
Grunting
Hair tossing, twisting, or sucking
Head banging, or jerking
Hissing
Hitting self or others
Honking
Hopping
Humming
Jumping
Kicking
Kissing self or others
Laughing at nothing funny
Licking objects or lips
Lip smacking
Misc. Noises

Moaning
Mouth open
Nail biting
Nose twitching
Nose wrinkling
Picking
Pinching
Pouting
Puffing
Pulling clothes, objects, or hair
Reflex inhibition
Repeating parts of words
Repeating phrases, or words
Rolling eyes
Scratching
Screaming
Shivering
Shoulder shrugging
Shouting
Skipping or Skipping steps
Smelling hands or objects
Snapping
Sniffing
Snorting
Spitting
Sucking
Squeaking
Squealing
Squinting
Stomping

Stuttering
Talking to oneself
Tearing things
Throat clearing
Throwing things
Touching objects
Twirling in circles
Walking on shoes
Walking on toes
Yelling-screaming
Yelping

Tics can increase in frequency and severity for a few weeks to a month or so, then start to subside. Children can experience more than one tic at a time. Following the disappearance of the first tic or tics, a few months may go by and then the same tic may re-emerge or a new tic may appear.

Chapter 4

Other Disorders and Behaviors Associated with Tourette's Syndrome

Not all people with Tourette's syndrome have disorders other than tics. However, many experience additional problems such as obsessive compulsive behavior, attention deficit disorder, or other mood disorders such as bipolar, sleep disorders, learning disorder, or aggressive behavior.

Obsessions consist of repetitive unwanted or bothersome thoughts.

Compulsive behaviors occur when a person feels that something must be done over and over and/or in a certain way. This could include touching an object with one hand after touching it with the other, to "even things up." Children sometimes beg their parents to repeat a sentence many times until it sounds right to them.

Attention Deficit Disorder With or Without Hyperactivity (ADD or ADHD)

This disorder occurs in many people with TS. Children may show signs of hyperactivity before TS symptoms appear. Symptoms of ADHD may include: difficulty with concentration, needing a great deal of supervision, always fidgeting/moving, moving from one activity to another without completion, failing to finish what is started, not listening, easily distracted, low impulse control.

Learning disabilities may include reading, and writing difficulties, problems with mathematics, and perceptual problems.

Difficulties with impulse control may include aggressive behavior and/or socially inappropriate acts.

Sleep disorders are fairly common among people with TS. These include frequent awakenings or walking or talking in one's sleep.

The wide range of behavioral symptoms that accompany tics may in fact be more disabling than the tics themselves. Patients, families, and physicians need to determine which set of symptoms is most disabling so that appropriate medications and therapies can be selected.

Because most symptoms do not impair most patients, the majority of Touretters require no medication. However, medication is available to help with symptoms that interfere with functioning and quality of life. The available TS medications are only able to help reduce specific symptoms.

The medication can help reduce the frequency and intensity of the tic symptoms. Medications are available to treat some of the associated behavioral disorders; although somewhat effective, they have also been known to increase tics. Many people can live with the tics; however, the associated behavior disorders are generally the symptoms that patients choose medication for.

Chapter 5

What We Wish We Knew with the Diagnosis of Tourette's Syndrome

It has been six months now since we received the diagnosis of Tourette's syndrome. Although it has been a huge relief, it has also been a huge adjustment. We had to redefine what was appropriate discipline for Dyllon, and what was the best way to get our point across.

We have found that Dyllon is easily frustrated when he can't explain himself. What works for us is patience, understanding, routine, and time.

For Dyllon, the diagnosis of Tourette's syndrome came with a diagnosis of bipolar disorder. He is easily frustrated, and if we don't intervene quick enough a rage will definitely be on the horizon. We worked out a simple system for simple tasks such as chores and homework. We call it the outline system. For most children, the simple task of cleaning their room is easy. For children of Tourette's and bipolar, the simple task of cleaning their room can be daunting. Outline what needs to be done. Start with pick up your clothes, then pick up your toys, make your bed, and so on. We have found that if we break down a chore into steps, it is easier to follow, and does not allow for the frustration to set in.

Set guidelines for behavior, and what the consequences will be. Give warnings, reminders, that one more time, and this will happen, and stick to it.

For us, consistency is the best policy. Have a regular routine that you follow: dinner time, showers, homework, etc. Routine goes a long way to keeping order in their head. They know what to expect every day at a given time. If the child is on medication, make sure you stick to the scheduled times. Get a pill box that you can take with you if you're out. Make a chart if need be, to check off times that medication is given. For me, I have been doing medication for a long time, and know the doses and scheduled times like a road map. It became second nature for me.

Know your child's tics, and how frequent they come on, their pattern, and what can trigger a new tic. This will help you decipher when one is going away, and another may possibly be coming. I know for us, when Dyllon's tics go away, I mean completely, something is about to happen. For instance, Dyllon's tics went away, and he started becoming more agitated, easily frustrated, and argumentative. His school work became messy, and attitude just plain stunk. Well this went on for four days, and on the fifth day, he was complaining of an earache. We made an appointment, and he had a double ear infection. Two days on an antibiotic, he was doing better, and what do you know, the tics came back. However this time it was a new tic he had never had before. He would talk very, very loud. That tic went away two weeks later, and his “old”tics came back. This time he had three at one time. That’s okay; he even recognized that a tic he had a few months ago was back.

Children are little wonders of amazement; they are so much more in tune with what is going on with them than we tend to give them credit for.

We were very fortunate from the get go to have wonderful doctors and teachers. The most important thing I can’t stress enough is have a psychologist and psychiatrist that you and your child are comfortable with. That in itself makes all the difference.

Chapter 6

Education Needs of Children with Tourette's Syndrome

Many children with disabilities find homework to be a challenge and source of stress. A good rule of thumb is to have clear and open communication with your child's teacher. If they know your child's issues at the beginning of the school year, you can avoid problems and stress early on. There are several things you can do to ensure a good start to the school year, and your child will thrive from them.

1. Establish a set routine at the beginning of the year. This may include when your child goes to bed during the school week. Establish when he/she is to do homework, and decide together where that should be. That location should be free of distraction.

2. Arrange a meeting with your child's teacher before school starts to discuss your child and TS. Many educators

only have a brief overview of Tourette's. Discuss things that help your child learn. Discuss any accommodations that they might need. Ask the teacher if a daily schedule is posted in a clearly visible spot. Ask to see if a card listing the daily schedule and times can be taped to the child's desk if one is not clearly posted. Express to your child's teacher that consistency is a great mood stabilizer for your child. Discuss the possibility of having your child's desk near the teacher's, for frequent refocusing if needed. Establish the use of private signals to signal behavior, so there is no public embarrassment. Find out what the policy is for students who need to leave the classroom. Do they have to ask permission, or do they have their own permanent pass, to avoid disrupting the class.

3. Some of the medications your child may be on may have the side effect of dehydration. Find out the policy of having a bottle of water in the classroom, or establish that frequent trips to the water fountain may be needed. Explain the side effects of your child's medication to their teacher, so they are aware of what to expect. For instance, Dyllon's medication makes him tired. Sometimes Dyllon will put his head down when his work is completed, or stay inside during recess for a quick cat nap. Dyllon's teacher allows him to do this, and will wake him when it is time to start something new, or when recess is over.

4. If your child has significant motor tics, arrange for their desk to be placed in such a manner that they have plenty of room.

5. Above all, have a good communication relationship with your child's teacher. I am in contact with mine through

phone and email. Most schools have internal email for their employees, so there should not be a huge problem in obtaining it to communicate.

6. Most school policy dictates that if your child takes medicine during the school hours, that a nurse must administer it. This is good policy. However, keep in mind that you don't have to make Tourette's syndrome a permanent part of your child's school record. Jason and I elected not to make it a part of his permanent record; however, everyone in the school that needs to know does.

Children with Tourette's syndrome are not different than any other child with or without disabilities. They all need a warm and nurturing environment in which to thrive. Consistency and routine are great ways to ensure your child has a successful academic experience.

Chapter 7

Medication Side Effects

Dealing with medication side effects in or out of the classroom setting is something we as parents will always deal with. Knowing what to expect from the medication your child is taking, or knowing that a switch to a new medication may take some time to adjust to a therapeutic level, is half the battle in dealing with side effects. We have been very fortunate that Dyllon has not experienced a lot of side effects, mainly tiredness. He has learned that when we try adjusting his medication or try another medication, in about a week or so, his body adjusts to the tiredness and he feels better. What we have come to do is give the bulk of his medication at night. He sleeps well, and is not so tired in the morning and can function through school without falling asleep an hour into the school day. Talk to your respective doctors about this, but we have found that it works best for us.

Chapter 8

Not Everything Is a Bed of Roses

It has been two years now since Dyllon was diagnosed with Tourette's, and things have not been great. Remember I said that consistency and routine were key factors to helping your child? Well, sometimes life does not allow for total consistency and routine.

My husband's child from his first marriage came to live with us a year ago, and life was not "normal" and calm like we had been adjusted to. Life became terrible. Dyllon does not do well with change, and this was a major change for him. His tics stopped completely, his rages came back stronger than ever, and once again we were asking ourselves what are we going to do to help him. You guessed it, more medication, another medication, and the waiting game to see if things would get better.

Dyllon likes for things to be fair, equal, and for everyone to be honest and nice. Well, in a perfect world that would be great; however, we don't live in a perfect world. His stepbrother would lie, steal, cheat, you name it, all the things we did not approve of, and all the things that drove Dyllon crazy with anger. Dyllon would get so angry when his brother would lie and do things to get him in trouble. Even though Dyllon was not at fault, and did not get in trouble, he still was angry and having rages over someone else's issues.

There was four months of school left, and we thought if we can just get through the end of the school year, summer will be here, and maybe things will get better. Again we were wrong. Things got worse.

Summertime came and the problems got more intense and the rages were more intense, the tics were back, but not in full force like usual. We were making routine trips to see the doctors, and making all sort of medication changes. We made it through the summer, and schooltime was here. I have to be honest and say I couldn't be happier. That meant routine, and consistency as far as the day went.

The smell of fall coming in goes hand in hand with new folders and glue. The sweet smell of a new school year. Dyllon was excited to start back, make new friends, and see some old ones. We went in early before school officially started to meet his teacher and discuss Tourette's with her. Believe it or not teachers do not know everything, as we would hope. His new teacher was nice and very welcoming of the information. We relayed to her different things that help Dyllon calm down, and put out the fire before a rage started.

The first week you would think would be a happy time of settling back into the swing of things, and meeting new people. Well for Dyllon it was not such a happy time. The stress was getting to him, and every day he would come home in tears. We tried to talk to him about things, and it was clear that Dyllon was not happy. He became depressed and dreaded going to school. We told him to give it some time, that it was his first week back, and things will get better. But they didn't. They got worse.

One morning Dyllon got up and was in tears; he did not want to go to school. I told him he could stay home, but we were going to talk and he had to tell us what was going on, and why he didn't want to go to school. After calming him down and calling Daddy to come home from work to have this discussion, he finally opened up. Dyllon began to open up about his feelings, and it broke my heart. He told us that kids were making fun of him, calling him names, tripping him in the hall, all the things you never want to have your child experience, especially your child with Tourette's. He was being called tic boy, weirdo, crazy, retarded, moron, jerky, and spazo. He explained that he felt stressed out and sad that kids were making fun of him, and lunch monitors were punishing him for not sitting still and being disruptive. He tried to explain to them that he has Tourette's, but to no avail. He asked, "Why can't I stay home and you teach me? I will learn from you. I will do what you ask me to." He was begging not to have to go back to school. We explained to him that we needed to discuss it, and talk with Regan and Mark about it and figure out if that would be the best solution for him. So we did just that, we talked to his doctors, and discussed the pros and cons of home schooling and came to the conclusion that if it was going to be less stress on

Dyllon, then that is what we needed to do, even if it was a temporary situation. We pulled him out the second week of school and he hasn't been back.

The decision of home schooling concerned Dyllon's father a lot; he wanted to make sure he still had social interaction to develop those social skills that every child needs to develop. Dyllon was already involved in church activities, and he had one friend in our neighborhood that didn't make fun of him and knew all about Tourette's. He asked Dyllon if we could explain it to him, and ever since they have been close friends. They don't see each other as much, but still play together and have sleepovers all the time.

Dyllon adjusted to home schooling very well. His attitude changed a bit, but you could still tell he was depressed. So again it was another medication change, and another period of adjustment. It is always hard to watch your child suffer when you know there is not one thing you can do to help. Reassurance and patience is a good policy, they will bounce back.

Chapter 9

Things Are Looking Up

We are in the fourth month of home schooling, and Dyllon is doing very well. We have the flexibility to schedule his learning hours around the times when he needs to take a nap, and dive in deeper to subjects that are interesting to him. That part of life is going well.

Remember, we had a major change take place in our family, a new child and sibling. It has been a year since this change, and the other part of life still was not great for Dyllon. He was still unstable, a lot of outbursts, but not full-on rages. They were few and far between but he was walking on that line of having one. We were having so many problems with Jason's other child that it was beginning to not only stress out Dyllon but us as well. That combination did not make life easy for anyone in our house. We made the decision that Jason's son had to go back and live with his mother. He wanted to go back and live with his mother, and so the plans were made to make that happen. When we told Dyllon of what was happening, it was like the gates of the tic waters opened up and we needed to hang on.

When Dyllon found out that his stepbrother was moving away, all the stress and anxiety that had been pent up for a year was released, not little by little, but all at once. The tics were back on in full force, three at a time, and vocal tics, some new ones we had never experienced before. They would last for two or three days, and go away and a new one would start. I saw my little boy smile again. I saw the twinkle in his eyes. I knew that things were going to be better, and they have been. Don't get me wrong, we still have hurdles, but they are small hills and not the big mountains we were experiencing. It will take some time for Dyllon's body to level out and settle into a "normal" tic pattern, but for now we have hope, where a year ago there was none.

Life is back to normal—well, what normal is for us, we are there. Christmas is around the corner in two weeks, and we have new hope for the next year. Dyllon is excelling in his studies and socially, and for now, life is calm.

What I want parents to know, if you're reading this book, that it helps you. That it gives you all the information we didn't have, when we needed it. I hope that you can sit back and realize that you are not alone, and that someone has been where you are, or might be.

I hope that you can learn from our mistakes and from our successes. I don't claim to be an expert on Tourette's, I do however claim to be a parent that has been there, and that has learned from trial and error. I hope that you will finish reading this book and know that your child with Tourette's is as normal as the child two doors down. That you are not in this alone, and that GOD has blessed you with this perfect child. Tourette's does not have to change your life or the quality of life for your child; it makes it better.

For now, we are home schooling, and life is great. We still have our ups and downs, but that is life. For us, we are a family that has a child with Tourette's. Tourette's does not have us.

Chapter 10

Things to Remember

Tourette's syndrome, like all disabilities, is a learning process. You will have periods of great enjoyment and periods of great heartache. It is up to you how you choose to make your way through it. The key is communication and consistency and give yourself a break.

Communicate with your doctor, communicate with your spouse, your family and friends. If you're having a bad day tell them. Be honest. No one expects you to be perfect, so don't pretend everything is alright when it is not. If you're feeling stressed out because of the many different things going on with your child, just saying it out loud can take the weight of the world off your shoulders.

Remember that your spouse is going through this as well, so when they need to yell, scream, cry, let them do it without judgement. If they need a little break, let them go. Have morning or nightly discussions with your spouse to discuss progress or issues with new ideas. Allow each other to speak, and hear each other out, and between the two of you come to a compromise. Remember you're in this together, so don't fight each other on issues.

Communication with your child's doctor is also vital. A parent's instinct is always the best. You know your child better than anyone. If you feel something is not quite right, wether it is with their mood, medication, side effects, whatever, call. A good psychiatrist or psychologist will welcome the call and give you ideas to try or reassure you that all is well. Sometimes reassurance is all we need to get through a small crisis.

Communication with your family is important, because they are the ones you can rely on and count on to give you a much-deserved break. Sometimes just a quick trip to the grocery store without the children can do wonders for your energy and self-awareness. Count on them, rely on them and when family members say we will watch the kids for a couple of hours, take them up on it. Go have a grown-up dinner, watch a movie, sit in the park and have a picnic, whatever you choose to do, just do it. I learned this lesson the hard way; you may not feel like you need a break, but as soon as you're out of the house and relaxing for a while, your brain kicks in and lets you know you are in overdrive, and you're gonna crash soon if you don't slow down. If you crash, what good are you to your child who needs you if you can't function because of the stress and lack of energy. My husband's favorite saying is "You're not supermom, you can't do it all and I love you for trying, but you're gonna break if you don't let someone help you." He was and is right when he says it now, but I will never admit to that again! So take the breaks when they are offered!

Consistency is the final key to maintaining sanity. Your special-needs child will thrive better in an environment where they know what to expect. Dinner is always at the same time. If your child has a favorite theme for their cups and plates, buy a couple of sets and always use them. If they like having three forks, so foods don't touch and mix, give them three forks. I think you get the idea. I learned it is better to pick my battles, and quite frankly these are very small. If simple things like three forks and the same plate make your child comfortable, do it. If your child has a favorite blanket, keep two on hand so that when one is being washed you have a backup. If that is not possible, make sure you can wash it and dry it so it is available the same day. This will cause less stress for your child and ultimately for you. Try to stick with the same detergents and fabric softeners; they will be able to tell if you switch, and won't take to it very well. If making some accommodations helps your child maintain low stress levels, do it. Not only will it be beneficial for them, but for you as well. When your child knows what comes next, or knows that he gets three forks, whatever the case may be, the happier they are.

Routine and consistency are always the best policy. Yes, there are times when a certain routine can't be followed, but you will learn to adapt and overcome. In these cases reassurance can go a long way to making them understand that it's okay. As for me and my family, we continue to strive to seek the best medical attention possible for Dyllon. With a new diagnosis of autism this year, we are constantly learning and trying to pave the way through this new disability, but that is yet another book to come.

I hope that you have received some helpful tips and insights in this book. I strived to incorporate all the things we had to learn the hard way, so that your journey would be a little easier. Not to say that any journey is easy when you're dealing with a special-needs child, but that maybe your journey is made a little easier through what we have learned.

Communicate, be consistent, and most importantly, take a break when you need it! I wish you well on your path, and when the time comes and it will, pay forward your insight and experience, as I will continue to do, so that another family's journey may be made a little easier.

Printed in the United States
129018LV00006B/463/A

9 781604 412758